The Plant-Based Diet For Beginners

Tailor Made Program To A Healthy, Fat-Free

Lifestyle With Simple, Quick And Tasty Recipes

And A Meal Plan To Reset & Energize Your Body

Amy Instant

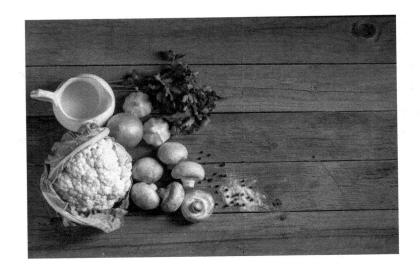

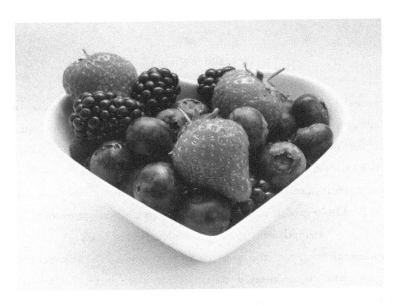

Table of Contents

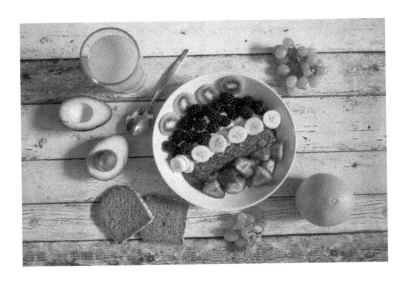

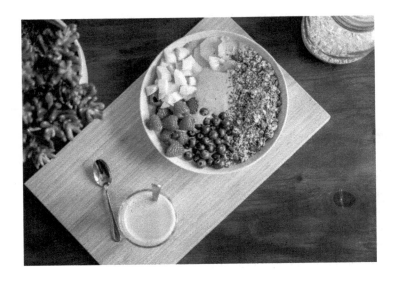

Introduction

Plant-based diet can vary from one person to another. However, the foundational idea is that we try to avoid processed food as much as possible and choose to use what we receive from the beautiful planet that we live in. By that, I mean the incredible ingredients derived from the earth. In essence, plant-based diet comes with a few benefits. Plant-based diet avoids using processed foods as much as possible. There are no animal products in the diet. The categories that are majorly included are vegetables, fruits, seeds and nuts, legumes, whole grains, and herbs and spices. The diet tries to limit the use of sugar, wheat-flour, and oil as much as possible. It focuses on the quality of food, mostly utilizing locally or farm-produced organic foods An important thing to remember here is that there are minimally processed foods included in the plant-based diet, such as non-dairy milk, tofu, and whole-wheat paste, to name a few. Overall, we aim to keep processed foods where they belong: on supermarket shelves, not in our refrigerators. When people look at the list of foods that come in a plant-based diet, they are often focused on how little we have to work on. However, that is probably due to the fact that many of the meat options have suddenly been removed. It feels as though a major part of the diet has been excluded due to it. How can life be fun without a nice steak? What can we do without chicken wings? Is there anything that can be done without a delicious fish? In reality, there are numerous ingredients that you can work with. Additionally, the fun is not just in the ingredients but how we prepare them. The growing demand has seen a rise in people trying out new recipes and mashing up ingredients in interesting ways. Have you heard of smoothies that contain cayenne pepper? Sounds pretty exciting, doesn't it? We are going to look at such wonderful and delicious recipes along with so many more dishes that use wholesome and natural ingredients. Some people are doing it; some people are talking about it, but there is still a lot of confusion about what a whole plant-based diet actually entails. Since we split food into their macronutrients: sugars, proteins, and fats, most of us are uncertain about nutrition. What if we were able to put these macronutrients back together again in order to free your mind from confusion and stress? The secret here is simplicity.

Plant Based Diet
A plant-based diet is a diet that comprises lots of products from plants, and very little or no amounts of animal products and processed foods.

Why plant-based diet?

Research suggests that those eating a plant-based diet tend to have a lower Body Mass Index (BMI) and therefore are slimmer, healthier and more energetic. Additionally, this means they tend to have lower rates of diabetes, heart disease and stroke than those who eat diets based around meat, especially processed meats.

This may be because plant-based foods such as fresh vegetables, fruits and nuts tend to be higher in complex carbs and fiber so keep you feeling fuller for longer. When you're full, you're far less likely to reach for unhealthy foods that won't nourish your body or mind.

They're also high in antioxidant, vitamins and minerals which are in a natural state and so more readily absorbed by the body.

Additionally, a plant-based diet has been shown to help reduce cholesterol, reduce high blood pressure and even certain types of cancer.

Types of Plant-Based Diet

Vegan: Diet includes vegetables, seeds, nuts, legumes, grains, and fruit and excludes all animal products (i.e. no animal flesh, dairy, or eggs). There are variations within the vegan diet as well such as the fruitarian diet made up mainly of fruits and sometimes nuts and seeds and the raw vegan diet where food is not cooked.

Vegetarian: Diet includes vegetables, fruit, nuts, legumes, grains, and seeds and excludes meat but may include eggs or dairy. The Ovo-lacto vegetarian diet incorporates dairy and eggs while the Ovo-vegetarian diet incorporates eggs and excludes dairy and the lacto vegetarian diet incorporates dairy but excludes eggs.

Semi-vegetarianism: Diet is mostly vegetarian but also incorporates some meat and animal products. The macrobiotic diet is a type of semi-vegetarian diet that emphasizes vegetables, beans, whole grains, naturally processed foods, and may include some seafood, meat, or poultry. The pescatarian diet includes plant foods, eggs, dairy, and seafood but no other types of animal flesh. People who subscribe to a semi-vegetarian diet sometimes describe themselves as flexitarians as well.

Difference between plant-based diet and vegan, vegetarian diet

A plant-based diet is all about easy healthy plant food option that includes fruits, vegetables, lentils, beans, and more. Other than the hardcore plant diet options, it allows the intake of low-fat dairy products that includes low-fat milk, low-fat cottage, mozzarella and cheddar cheese as well. Having a plant-based diet doesn't require that you avoid all the animal-based products.

A vegan diet states that one should eat all the vegetables and avoid any meat products. It is simply that a person prefers eating vegetables and fruits instead of meat and other fats. Vegan culture involves not using any other animal products not in food nor any daily use.

A vegetarian diet is about focusing on plant foods but also eating animal products such as honey and milk. The main difference with veganism is that vegans avoid any form of animal products while vegetarians do not eat meat but they eat animal products like honey and milk.

Benefits of a Plant-Based Diet

•   Environmentally friendly: Plant-based diet is all environmentally friendly. When masses are following the plant-based diet that means there will be more plants and no more packing food. No processed or packaged food means there won't be any disposal or trash out there. On the other hand, more plants will provide more oxygen for people and give them nutrients through food. It is an overall a good package for the ultimate healthy and happy society.

• Better organ health: Plant-based diet is good for not only a specific organ like liver, heart or kidneys, but it helps your overall body to have a perfect mechanism. It gives proper attention to all the organs and make it possible for a person to have the best of health in any manner. Other than organs, the diet helps to increase muscular strength, make bones stronger, hair longer and many more. It is all about how you are managing the diet and you will be able to get the best results within a few days of starting with it.

• Benefits beyond health: The benefits of plant-based diet are not limited to the health and fitness only. It is a complete package of ultimate benefits that prolong in society and help each aspect of the society to grow better. Since the diet is all about plants, it means one needs to have fresh vegetables and fruits available in surroundings. Moreover, it enhances the consumption and utilization of all the products and bi-products. Here are some of the value-added benefits of the plant-based diet that is commendable:

• Lowers Blood Pressure: One of the reasons why plant-based foods contribute to low blood pressure is that they tend to have high amount of potassium, which in turn helps you manage your blood pressure (Physicians Committee for Responsible Medicine, n.d.). Additionally, potassium has also been known to reduce anxiety and stress. Now, guess what meat has little of? That's right. Potassium. Some foods that have a high amount of potassium are fruits, whole grains, nuts, and legumes.

• Prevents Chronic Diseases: Obesity? Cancer? Diabetes? These are illnesses that you can avoid or minimize the risk of with a plant-based diet. People who are already suffering from chronic diseases are asked to live on plant-based food because they help improve lifespans (Nordqvist, 2012).

• Lowers Blood Sugar Levels: One thing that plant-based diets are rich in is fiber. When you consume fiber, your body reduces the amount of sugar it absorbs into the bloodstream. Additionally, fiber does not make you feel hungry really fast. When you do not feel full, you end up consuming more food than necessary. Plant-based foods help prevent such a situation from arising.

• Ideal for Weight Loss: When you are consuming a plant-based diet, you are cutting down on excess fats and maintaining a healthy level of weight. You don't even have to worry about calorie restrictions! Weight loss is possible with a plant-based diet simply because of the fiber we mentioned previously. It helps you manage your hunger, and you also receive the necessary amount of minerals, proteins, and vitamins from your green meal.

• Saves Time and Money: Plant-based foods are not as difficult to prepare as meat-based foods. In fact, you will take less time to prepare an organic meal. When you really need, you can easily put together some healthy ingredients and make a quick salad. Furthermore, you spend less money by preparing food using plant-based ingredients. When you source local and organic products, you end up shelling out less cash for the items that you would like to buy.

• Lowers Cholesterol Level: This might sound like a myth, but plants contain no cholesterol. Even if you pick out coconut and cocoa plants, they do not contain any cholesterol. Hence, when you are at risk of having a high level of cholesterol, a plant-based diet will help you bring it back down to a much healthier level.

Plant -Based Diet Blue Print

Foods to Eat

Vegetables: tomatoes, cauliflower, spinach, carrots, kale, asparagus, peppers, and broccoli.

Whole Grains: rolled oats, quinoa, pastas made with brown rice, barley, faro, and brown rice, wild rice, amaranth, buckwheat, spelt, kamut, and couscous.

Legumes: chickpeas, peanuts, black beans, peas, and lentils.

Fruits: citrus fruits, bananas, apples, pineapples, berries, and pears.

Starchy Vegetables: sweet potatoes, squash, regular potatoes.

Healthy Fats: avocados, unsweetened coconut, olive oils, and coconut oils.

Seeds: Nut Butters, and Nuts: Macadamia nuts, sunflower seeds, pumpkin seeds, almond butter, cashews, almonds, and tahini.

Plant-Based Milks: almond milk, coconut milk, cashew milk. For this category, it might be tempting to get the sweetened varieties to help you get accustomed to the taste. Initially, that is okay, however, for the long-term, the sweeteners in these milks are not great for your overall health. Perhaps eventually, you can experiment with making some great nut-milk at home, where you can control how much it's sweetened.

Spices and Seasonings: rosemary, turmeric (this spice in particular is great for reducing internal inflammation), curry, sea salt, basil, black pepper.

Drinks: unsweetened coffees and teas, fresh fruit and vegetable juices or smoothies, plain water, sparkling water. There are some great new brands of flavored and sparkling waters available that are sugar-free and help abstain from pop and sweetened juice. No matter what diet you choose, drinking loads of water is great for your body. Additionally, if you really want to boost your immunity and also help your body detox naturally, try adding some berries, sliced orange/lemon/cucumber, mint or lavender to your water. They each make for a tasty flavored water combination either altogether or individually as well.

Condiments: mustard, vegan mayonnaise, soy sauce, tamari, vinegar (apple cider vinegar is wonderful), lemon juice, salsa, and nutritional yeasts.

Plant-based Proteins: tempeh and tofu. A little later, we will provide fabulous recipes for these meatless, yet protein packed, plant-based options.

Foods to Avoid

Animal Foods

Yes, no duh! Being plant-based means that you should avoid animal foods as much as possible. Whether you are doing this for health purposes or for the love of animals, just be sure you try to avoid animal products as much as possible. Some of the more popular options include

Meat: Organs, Veal, Pork, Lamb, and Beef, etc.

Poultry: Duck, Goose, Turkey, Chicken, etc.

Eggs: Any Type of Egg

Dairy: Ice Cream, Butter, Cheese, Yogurt, etc.

Seafood and Fish: All Fish, Lobster, Crab, Mussels, Shrimp, etc.

Bee Products: Honey, Royal Jelly, etc.

Animal Derived Ingredients & Additives: This is where it can get a bit tricky when it comes to living a plant-based diet. One moment you are enjoying one of your favorite snacks, the next you are reading the label and realizing it has an ingredient that has been derived from an animal. Of course, we all make mistakes, but by being educated, you can avoid this mistake in the first place!

Tips to Get Started

As a newbie to plant-based diets, you should understand that this is not something you can just jump into. Your body needs time to adapt to the new style of eating. As you take this important step in your life, here are a few pointers to help you get started.

Find Your Motivation

Before making any changes to your diet, it is essential to take a step back and determine the reasons why you need to make this step. Why do you want to try a plant-based diet? Maybe you are suffering from a disease and this is the best strategy for you to reduce the effects of the disease. Alternatively, it could be that you are looking for a way of improving your health as a means to your overall happiness. Good health means a good heart. It doesn't matter what reasons you have for taking this path. What you need to do is write down your motivation and remind yourself of it every time you wake up.

Start Slow

This is the second most important consideration you should bear in mind. You need to initiate your transition slowly. Select a few foods that are plant-based and begin rotating them for about a week. A good tip here is to select foods that you often enjoy. They can range from lentil stew, oatmeal, jacket potatoes, beans, or veggie stir-fry. Human beings are creatures of habit. Therefore, make a list of the most common plant-based foods that interest you. This should be your starting point as you help your body make a smooth transition.

Cut Down on Processed Foods and Meat

A slow transition guarantees that your body adapts well to the change in diet. In line with this, you shouldn't just avoid processed foods and meat from the get-go. This should be done gradually. Begin by cutting down on your meat intake. Increase the portions of veggies on your plate while reducing the meat portions. After some time, get rid of them entirely as you will have gained the perception that you can do without them. Later on, work on your recipes. If you were a huge fan of beef chili, you can swap the meat with portobello mushrooms. The idea is to continue eating your favorite meals, but as a plant-based version of what you used to have.

Try a Plant-Based Breakfast

After making a few attempts here and there, your next step should be to grab a plant-based meal every day. It would be a good idea for you to start your morning with a vegetarian breakfast. Maybe you are worried that you don't know where to start. There are several plant-based recipes for breakfast, lunch, and dinner that will be provided in this guide. They should help you get started on adopting a plant-based lifestyle.

Surround Yourself with Wholesome Foods

If you are going to adopt a healthy lifestyle, then it is important that you surround yourself with healthy foods. In this case, no other forms of food will be okay; you should only have plant-based foods. Walk around your kitchen as you try and evaluate whether the foods around you are helpful to your goal. If not, don't hesitate to throw them away or donate them. Just because you bought them doesn't imply that you will be wasting food if you choose not to eat them.

Watch Your Protein Portions

The Dietary Reference Intake recommends that the average amount of protein that the body needs is about 0.8 grams per kilogram of body weight. This implies that the typical, sedentary man will require about 56 grams of daily protein intake, whereas a woman will require about 46 grams (Gunnars, 2018). This shows that we only need a fraction of our protein intake to supplement the body with what it needs. Unfortunately, most dieters over-consume proteins with the idea that the body requires the nutrients. What we forget is that too much of something can be toxic and dangerous.

Whether the body needs it or not, watching our portions is vital. While striving to live on a plant-based diet, you should be careful of the amounts of protein you consume. Excessive intake will undeniably lead to negative health effects. What you need to do is make sure that your plant foods have enough calories to provide your body with the energy it needs for metabolism and other purposes.

Educate Yourself

In addition to focusing on food, you should also invest your time and money in educating yourself, just like you are doing by reading this book. It is unfortunate that digital media and advertising has polluted our minds. We are blinded from realizing that plant-based foods are the best foods for our bodies and the planet we live on. Educating yourself is the surest way to get the answers to lifestyle-related questions. You should recognize that, by taking the time to learn, you will be motivated to focus on your goal since you know what you are after.

Find Like-Minded People

Relating to like-minded individuals will be helpful in good and bad times. These are people who are also looking to benefit from eating plant-based foods. Therefore, by relating to them, you can share success stories as well as help each other out in times of need. With the advent of the Internet, it should not be difficult for you to find other people who are vegetarians. Browse through social media pages and join their groups. Here, you will find significant information about your new diet plan. For instance, some people will be eager to share tasty, plant-based recipes with you.

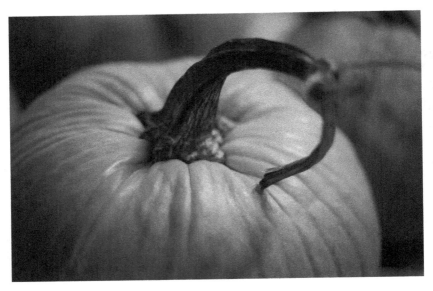

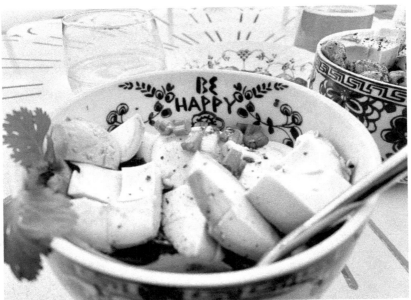

Health Benefits Of The Plant-based Diet

The primary objective of a healthy, plant-based diet is to minimize the consumption of animal foods, eggs, dairy products, oils, and processed foods while maximizing the consumption of plant foods that are full of needed nutrients. The diet encourages the inclusion of fruits, raw and cooked vegetables, peas, beans, soybeans, lentils, nuts, and seeds. The diet is generally low in fat while being high on the satiety scale, which means the food you eat will fill you up and keep you fuller for longer with fewer calories.

Plants are good for us because they are healthy. Vegetables and fruits are loaded with fiber, antioxidants, minerals, and vitamins. Most people do not regularly consume enough fiber, especially those whose diet is high in processed foods. But besides being full of vitamins and fiber, eating a plant-based diet has other health benefits that will keep you living healthier for longer.

Obesity

Obesity is a medical condition where a person is carrying around more weight than is healthy for them to carry on their bodies. Many people could stand to lose a few pounds, but an obese person has a higher body mass index (BMI) than most people. You will divide your weight in kilograms by your height in meters squared to find your body mass index. There are numerous online calculators that will determine your BMI for you. Generally, anything over twenty-five is considered overweight. If the BMI number is thirty or more, then the person is considered to be obese. Obesity can definitely increase your overall risk of developing many conditions, including high blood pressure, cardiovascular disease, and Type 2 Diabetes.

People become obese for many reasons. The number one cause of obesity is simply consuming too many calories. When you eat more calories than your body needs you to eat to provide energy for your body, then the excess food is stored as fat, and you become obese. Certain types of food are more likely to cause you to be obese, such as foods that are high in sugar and fat. These foods are high in sugar, which is very easy for the body to turn into glucose, or blood sugar, in your body.

When you eat food, your body begins breaking the food down into usable molecules as soon as you begin chewing. When the food reaches your stomach, it encounters various stomach acids that continue to break the food down into tiny particles. After that, the food particles pass into your intestines, where they are either absorbed as usable nutrients or eliminated as waste products. The food particles that are absorbed then move into your bloodstream as glucose, the blood sugar. This glucose is the fuel that the cells need in order to complete their processes and restore themselves. While your stomach was digesting the food, your pancreas was making insulin, which is the hormone the body needs in order to move the glucose into the cells. When the insulin has moved all of the glucose into the cells that the cells will accept, any leftover glucose will be stored as fat in your body. This is a normal function of the body, and it is leftover from the time when food sources were sometimes scarce and the body might not know when it would receive its next meal, so it developed the habit of storing a bit of food for the lean times. When you continuously eat more food, more calories than you need to consume then your body will store more leftover glucose as fat, and you will eventually become obese.

People who follow a plant-based diet weigh less than their meat-eating counterparts and are actually able to eat a larger amount of food. Three ounces of beef weighs in at 213 calories, while three ounces of carrots only has ninety calories. Three ounces of bell pepper gives you seventy-five calories, three ounces of celery is forty-five calories, and three ounces of cucumber brings in thirty calories. Add to this the fact that vegetables are high in fiber, which passes right through the body as a waste product, and it is easy to see how weight can be controlled by following a plant-based diet.

Metabolic Syndrome

Constantly overeating and being obese will eventually lead to metabolic syndrome. As you eat food, your body makes insulin in order to be able to move the product of the food being consumed, the glucose in your blood, into your cells. The insulin opens the doors of the cells to allow glucose to enter. When food is consumed continuously, or too much food is consumed, insulin is constantly being produced in order to deal with the steady stream of food flowing through the body. Eventually, the cells become full, and they stop responding to the prompt of the insulin. They will accept no more glucose from the blood. So the body has no choice but to store the glucose as fat in the body. This is known as insulin resistance and is one of the major factors in developing metabolic syndrome, which is characterized by having a large waist, from the fat stored underneath the skin, and will eventually lead to the development of life-threatening diseases.

The fiber-rich foods, which include vegetables, nuts, and seeds that are consumed on the plant-based diet, will help to guard against the development of the metabolic syndrome. Following the plant-based diet will lead to a lower weight which in turn will lead to lowered levels of fat and blood sugar. The followers of the plant-based diet will also have less digestive issues, which is another cause of metabolic syndrome.

High Blood Pressure

In monitoring your overall health, your blood pressure is an important number to know and try to control. There are two individual numbers that are used to measure your blood pressure. The first number, the number on top, is the systolic pressure. The second number, the number on the bottom, is the diastolic pressure. The systolic pressure is the measure of the amount of force, or pressure, which the walls of your arteries undergo when your heart muscle contracts to force the blood to move from the heart and out to the body. The diastolic number measures the amount of pressure that the moving blood puts on your arteries when your heart is resting. So if your heart muscle is working harder to force blood out to the arteries, then your blood pressure reading will be higher than is considered healthy.

High blood pressure is caused by the strain your heart produces, trying to move your oxygenated blood out to all of the cells in your body through the miles and miles of arteries and veins. As people gain weight, their bodies will produce more lengths of arteries and veins so that it is able to supply blood, oxygen, and other nutrients to all parts of your body. If your body did not do these things, then those extra parts of you, like the excess belly fat, would eventually die from starvation. But the body intends for you to keep all of your parts healthy, so it works harder to keep all of you well fed.

When the systolic reading is over 120 and the diastolic reading is over

80, a person is considered to be on their way to developing high blood pressure. Sometimes a reading will be higher if the person is stressed, sick, or has just drunk a hot beverage or smoked a cigarette. But when the reading is constantly higher, then high blood pressure is a real threat. Continuous high blood pressure can lead to kidney disease, strokes, heart problems, and loss of vision. Managing your intake of healthy foods in your daily diet is one of the best ways to naturally lower your high blood pressure. A balanced diet of healthy foods like vegetables, fruits, and whole grains is proven to lower overall body weight and, along with it, high blood pressure. Remember, if the heart does not need to pump blood through all those extra miles of arteries, it won't need to work as hard. And the plant-based diet will provide healthy alternatives to animal fat in the form of omega oil, nuts, and seeds. And foods that are higher in potassium, like bananas, mushrooms, beans, and tomatoes, are known to help lower high blood pressure.

Cardiovascular Disease

Cardiovascular disease refers to any illness or disease that happens in any part of the cardiovascular system, which is your lungs, arteries, veins, and heart. Most of the issues that involve the cardiovascular disease begin with high blood pressure and a condition known as atherosclerosis. This is a disease of the arteries in the body that is caused by deposits of fatty material known as plaque build-up on the inner walls of the arteries. Plaque buildup is a collection of excess bits of waste products, fat cells, and calcium deposits that collect along the inside walls of your arteries in spots that have become thinned from the force of high blood pressure. Plaque buildup is another thing that will cause the heart to pump faster and harder as it tries to push blood flow past these blockages.

An accumulation of plaque will slow and eventually block the flow of healthy blood through your body, which makes it more difficult for nutrients and oxygen to get to all parts of your body. Another concern involved with plaque buildup is that these formations can eventually break loose and allow little bits of debris to float through your bloodstream. If one of these bits of debris reaches the major arteries n your neck, the blockage could cause you to have a stroke. If one of these blockages reaches the arteries in your heart, then you could suffer a heart attack.

Blood cholesterol is another factor that will lead to good or bad cardiovascular health and is directly affected by your diet. Cholesterol is a wax type of substance that is produced by your liver that helps your body to produce hormones and build membranes for your cells. Your body will naturally produce the amount of cholesterol that it needs, so there is no need to consume excess amounts of cholesterol for the health of your body. When your cholesterol is measured, the doctor is looking at three separate numbers. The first number is your total cholesterol level, which measures the total level of cholesterol in your blood. The second number is the high-density lipoprotein (HDL) level, which is the measurement of the good cholesterol in your blood. The third number is the low-density lipoprotein (LDL) level, which measures the bad cholesterol in your blood. The LDL level is the amount of the bad type of fat that you have floating around in your blood, the type of fat that causes plaque in your arteries.

The benefit of the plant-based diet is that plants are naturally low in fat and contain very small amounts of saturated fat, no dietary cholesterol, and abundant amounts of natural fiber. Saturated fats and cholesterol, which are found in eggs, cheese, and meats, are major contributors to the accumulation of plaque deposits in the arteries, which will eventually lead to some form of cardiovascular disease. The high levels of potassium in plants will help to lower high blood pressure. The high fiber levels in plants will help to lower high blood cholesterol. The low amounts of cholesterol and saturated fats will no add to plaque buildup in the arteries. And the plant-based diet is known to help relieve inflammation, which can also lead to heart disease. And since plants are rich in their levels of soluble fiber, they help to lower the levels of cholesterol in the body by slowing the body's absorption of cholesterol and reducing the amount the liver naturally produces.

Adult-onset diabetes or sugar diabetes are just alternative titles for Type 2 Diabetes. Type 1 Diabetes, the one most often diagnosed in childhood, is caused by the pancreas stopping the production of insulin. For some as yet unknown reasons, the pancreas ceases to function, and the body no longer produces insulin to carry the blood glucose into the cells. Type 2 Diabetes is generally preventable, and the reason it is often referred to as sugar diabetes is from the belief that people who consume too much sugar will get diabetes. This is partially true because a diet of highly processed foods that are high in sugar is one of the premier causes of Type 2 Diabetes.

When your body begins to resist the good effects of the insulin, it produces you begin metabolic syndrome. Your pancreas will make enough insulin and secrete it into your bloodstream to take the appropriate amount of glucose to your cells for energy. The problem starts when there is an excess of glucose in your bloodstream. When the cells are full, then the insulin will store the excess glucose as fat, and then the levels of glucose will drop back to normal. When this finely tuned production is thrown off course by excess food consumption, which causes excess insulin production, which causes excess glucose storage, then the levels of glucose will build up in your bloodstream, and this is when the diagnosis of diabetes happens. Being overweight is the single largest risk factor for the development of diabetes. Inactivity and abdominal fat are also risk factors.

A plant-based diet is crucial for reducing the risk of developing Type 2 Diabetes. For the best levels of health, the consumption of animal protein should be minimized. The plant-based diet can reduce the risk of developing Type 2 Diabetes by lowering the risk of gaining excessive amounts of weight. People who consume a plant-based diet typically eat less fat and fewer calories. They also consume less cholesterol and saturated fats while consuming more potassium and fiber, all of which will help to prevent or eliminate Type 2 Diabetes.

Cancer is a somewhat broad term that describes what happens when changes in the cells cause abnormal growth and division. Cancer will cause cells to divide uncontrollably, which will result in the formation of tumors and damage to your immune system. Most of the cells in your body have fixed lifespans and specific functions. Cells will naturally die during the course of your life, and new cells will take its place. Cancer cells know how to grow, but they lack the elements that tell them when to stop growing and when to die. They continue to grow in the body and use up nutrients and oxygen that the body could use in better ways. Some cancers are born with us and will appear at some time in our life, and those can't be prevented. But some cancers are caused by poor nutrition and the effects of excess body weight.

Being overweight is directly linked to the development of several types of cancers, including cancers of the pancreas, esophagus, kidney, rectum and colon, liver, and gallbladder. Excess body fat leads to inflammation and suppressed immune system function. It will hamper the production of certain hormones like estrogen and insulin. Being obese interferes with proper cell growth and production. And it can adversely affect the way in which the body uses certain hormones.

People who are obese usually have higher levels of inflammation, which can cause cell damage and are associated with digestive diseases that can lead to cancer of the rectum and colon. Also, people who are obese generally eat less fiber than is recommended. Fiber cleanses the colon and rectum as the waste product passes through and leaves less behind that can cause inflammations and diseases. Excess fat in your body can lead to the production of gall stones, which could lead to the development of cancer of the gallbladder.

Plant foods are excellent sources of substances that are called phytochemicals, and these can lead to protection from cancer-causing cells. The pigments that give bright colors to vegetables and fruits are the same substances that will help you prevent or fight cancer. And plant food contains fiber, which removes excess waste material and hormones from your body.

Replacing the animal protein in your diet with plant-based protein will lower your risk of death from heart disease and cancer. Plant-based proteins from foods such as grains, legumes, and vegetables can improve overall weight, cholesterol levels, and blood pressure. People who consume a plant-based diet have lower body mass indexes. They are more successful at keeping excess weight off. A plant-based diet will lower your risk of high blood pressure and cardiovascular disease. Your blood sugar levels and cholesterol levels will be easier to control. Your levels of inflammation will be reduced. Your risk of developing diabetes will be reduced. You will greatly benefit by lowering the amounts of animal substances you take in and increasing your consumption of beneficial plant-based foods.

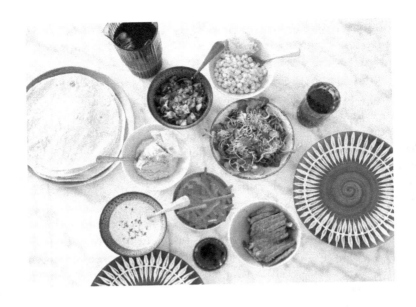

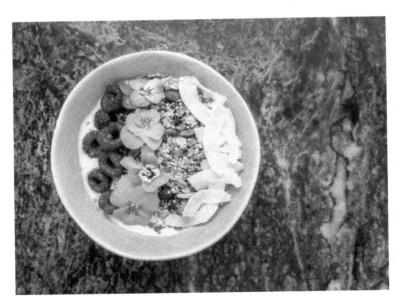

Chapter 1. Breakfasts

1. Corn Pudding

Preparation time: 10 minutes

Cooking time: 20 minutes

Servings: 2

Ingredients:

3 tbsp cornmeal

1 cup corn kernels

2 chopped shallots

1 cup coconut milk

1.5 cup water

Directions:

Prepare the Instant Pot using the sauté function.

Lightly spritz with the cooking spray and add the shallots. When softened, toss in the cornmeal, milk, and corn kernels.

Pour the contents into a baking dish and cover with foil.

Rinse out the pot. Pour water into the Instant Pot and add the trivet. Add the dish and close the lid.

Use the manual setting to cook for about 20 minutes.

Quick release the pressure and serve.

Nutrition:

Calories 170, Total Fat 4.4g, Total Carbohydrate 28.6g, Protein 4.4g

2. Maple & Vanilla Toast

Preparation time: 5 minutes

Cooking time: 2 minutes

Servings: 2

Ingredients:

2 tbsp maple syrup

1 tsp vanilla extract

2 bread slices

2 tbsp vegan butter

Directions:

Combine the vanilla and syrup to brush over the slices of bread—all sides.

Warm up the Instant Pot using the sauté function. Melt the butter and add the prepared bread slices.

Sauté the bead for two minutes on each side.

Serve with your favorite toppings.

Nutrition:

Calories 224, Total Fat 0.8g, Total Carbohydrate 25.3g, Protein 2.3g

3. Pomegranate Porridge

Preparation time: 5 minutes

Cooking time: 4 minutes

Servings: 4

Ingredients:

2 cups, oats

1.5 cups water

2 tbsp pomegranate molasses

1.5 cups pomegranate juice

Directions:

Pour all of the fixings into the Instant Pot. Stir well.

Secure the top and use the manual setting for 3-4 minutes using high pressure.

When ready, just quick release the pressure and serve.

Nutrition:

Calories 400, Total Fat 6g, Total Carbohydrate 63.7g, Protein 14g

4. Strawberry Oatmeal

Preparation time: 5 minutesCooking time: 3 minutes

Servings: 4

Ingredients:

2 cups rolled oats

1 handful chopped strawberries

4 cups water

1 tbsp maple syrup

2 tbsp flax meal

Directions:

Combine all the fixings in the Instant Pot. Stir well.

Secure the lid and start the cooker using the manual setting for 3 minutes on high.

Natural release the pressure for about 10 minutes. Quick release and serve.

Portion into the dishes and top with a few berries. Relax and enjoy.

Nutrition:

Calories 200, Total Fat 3g, Total Carbohydrate 25g, Protein 6g

5. Sweet Potato Toast

Preparation time: 10 minutes

Cooking time: 5 minutes

Servings: 4

Ingredients:

3 tbsp vegan butter

2 sweet potatoes

1 tsp turmeric powder

Directions:

Peel the potatoes and slice.

Warm up the Instant Pot using the sauté function. Add one tbsp of the butter. Add 1/3 of the slices into the pot and sauté until browned on each side.

Continue until all of the potatoes are done.

Sprinkle the toasts with the turmeric and garnish with your favorite toppings such as coconut cream and veggies.

Nutrition:

Calories 140, Total Fat 4g, Total Carbohydrate 27g, Protein 2.5g

6. Vanilla Quinoa

Preparation time: 5 minutes Cooking time: 1 minute

Servings: 3

Ingredients:

1 cup uncooked quinoa

2 cups water

1.5 tbsp maple syrup

2 tbsp cinnamon powder

1 tsp vanilla

1 pinch salt

Crushed almonds, cherries, fresh berries

Directions:

Add the quinoa, water, maple syrup, cinnamon powder, vanilla, and salt into the Instant Pot.

Set the pressure manually for 1 minute.

When done, let it do a natural release for 10 minutes. Then, quick release the remainder of the pressure and serve with toppings.

Nutrition:

Calories 280, Total Fat 4g, Total Carbohydrate 47g, Protein 9g

7. Baby Spinach Salad

Preparation time: 15 minutes

Cooking time: 0 minutes

Servings: 4

Ingredients:

1 bag baby spinach, washed and dried

1 red bell pepper, cut in slices

1 cup cherry tomatoes, cut in halves

1 red onion, finely chopped

1 cup black olives, pitted

1 tsp dried oregano 1 large garlic clove

3 tbsp red wine vinegar

4 tbsp olive oil

Salt and freshly ground black pepper, to taste

Directions:

Prepare the dressing by blending the garlic and the oregano with the olive oil and the vinegar in a food processor.

Place the spinach leaves in a large salad bowl and toss with the dressing. Add the rest of the ingredients and give everything a toss again. Season to taste with black pepper and salt.

Nutrients:

Calories 211, Fat 18.2g, Sodium 365g, Carb: 12.4g, Fiber: 4.7g, Sugar: 4.3g, Protein: 3.8g

8. Spanish Rice

Preparation time: 10 minutes

Cooking time: 20 minutes

Servings: 6

Ingredients:

1½ cups white rice, rinsed

1 small onion, peeled and chopped

1 ½ cups mixed bell pepper, diced

1 medium tomato, seeded and diced

6-ounce tomato paste

Directions:

Switch on the instant pot, grease the inner pot with 1 tablespoon olive oil, press the sauté/simmer button, then adjust cooking time to 5 minutes and let preheat.

Add onion, 1 teaspoon minced garlic and all the pepper, cook for 3 minutes, then season with ¾ teaspoon salt, ½ teaspoon red chili powder and ¼ teaspoon ground cumin, pour in 2 cups vegetable broth and stir until mixed.

Press the cancel button, secure instant pot with its lid in the sealed position, then press the manual button, adjust cooking time to 10 minutes, select high-pressure cooking and let cook until instant pot buzz.

Instant pot will take 10 minutes or more to build pressure, and when it buzzes, press the cancel button and do natural pressure release for 10 minutes or more until pressure knob drops down.

Then carefully open the instant pot, fluff the rice with a fork, sprinkle with parsley and serve.

Nutrition:

Calories 211, Total Fat 3.6g, Total Carbohydrate 41g, Protein 4.6g

9. Spiced Brown Rice

Preparation time: 10 minutes

Cooking time: 22 minutes

Servings: 3

Ingredients:

1 1/2 cups brown rice

1/2 cup chopped apricots, dried

1/2 cup cashews, roasted

1/2 cup raisins

Directions:

Switch on the instant pot, place all the ingredients in the inner pot, sprinkle with 2 teaspoons grated ginger, 1/2 teaspoon cinnamon and 1/8 teaspoon ground cloves, pour in 3 cups water and stir until mixed.

Secure instant pot with its lid in the sealed position, then press the manual button, adjust cooking time to 22 minutes, select high-pressure cooking and let cook until instant pot buzz.

Instant pot will take 10 minutes or more to build pressure, and when it buzzes, press the cancel button and do natural pressure release for 10 minutes or more until pressure knob drops down.

Then carefully open the instant pot, fluff the rice with a fork and garnish with cashews.

Serve straight away.

Nutrition:

Calories 216, Total Fat 2g, Total Carbohydrate 45g, Protein 5g

10. Salsa Brown Rice and Kidney Beans

Preparation time: 10 minutes

Cooking time: 25 minutes

Servings: 4

Ingredients:

1 1/2 cup brown rice, uncooked

1 1/4 cup red kidney beans, uncooked

½ bunch of cilantros, chopped

1 cup tomato salsa

Directions:

Switch on the instant pot, add brown rice and beans in the inner pot, pour in 2 cups water and 3 cups vegetable stock, then add salsa and chopped cilantro stems, don't stir.

Secure instant pot with its lid in the sealed position, then press the manual button, adjust cooking time to 25 minutes, select high-pressure cooking and let cook until instant pot buzz.

Instant pot will take 10 minutes or more to build pressure, and when it buzzes, press the cancel button and do natural pressure release for 10 minutes or more until pressure knob drops down.

Then carefully open the instant pot, stir the beans-rice mixture, garnish with cilantro and serve.

Nutrition:

Calories 218, Total Fat 4g, Total Carbohydrate 37g, Protein 10g

11. Walnut Lentil Tacos

Preparation time: 10 minutes

Cooking time: 25 minutes

Servings: 12

Ingredients:

1 cup brown lentils, uncooked

1 medium white onion, peeled and diced

15-ounce diced tomatoes, fire-roasted

3/4 cup chopped walnuts

Directions:

Switch on the instant pot, grease the inner pot with 1 tablespoon olive oil, press the sauté/simmer button, then adjust cooking time to 5 minutes and let preheat.

Add onion and ½ teaspoon minced garlic, cook for 4 minutes, then season with 1/2 teaspoon salt, 1/4 teaspoon ground black pepper, 1/4 teaspoon oregano, 1 tablespoon red chili powder, 1/2 teaspoon paprika, 1/4 teaspoon red pepper flakes, 1 1/2 teaspoon ground cumin and stir until mixed.

Pour in 2 ¼ cups vegetable broth, press the cancel button, secure instant pot with its lid in the sealed position, then press the manual button, adjust cooking time to 15 minutes, select high-pressure cooking and let cook until instant pot buzz.

Instant pot will take 10 minutes or more to build pressure, and when it buzzes, press the cancel button, do natural pressure release for 5 minutes and then do quick pressure release until pressure knob drops down.

Then carefully open the instant pot, stir the lentils, then spoon in the tortillas, top with lettuce and jalapeno and serve.

Nutrition:

Calories 157.5, Total Fat 4g, Total Carbohydrate 25g, Protein 6.5g

12. Lettuce Wraps with Spicy Tofu

Preparation time: 5 minutes

Cooking time: 5 minutes

Servings: 3

Ingredients:

1 banana

¼ cup rolled oats, or 1 scoop plant protein powder

1 tablespoon flaxseed, or chia seeds

1 cup raspberries, or other berries

1 cup chopped mango (frozen or fresh)

½ cup non-dairy milk (optional)

1 cup water

Directions:

Purée everything in a blender until smooth, adding more water (or non-dairy milk) if needed.

Add none, some, or all of the bonus boosters, as desired. Purée until blended.

Nutrition:

Calories 550, Total Fat 9g, Total Carbohydrate 116g, Protein 13g

13. Fried Seitan Finger

Preparation time: 15 minutes

Cooking time: 10 minutes

Servings: 4

Ingredients:

1 cup all-purpose flour

1 teaspoon garlic powder

1 teaspoon onion powder

pinch of cayenne pepper

1 teaspoon dried thyme

½ teaspoon sea salt

½ teaspoon freshly ground black pepper

1 cup soy milk

1 tablespoon lemon juice

2 tablespoons baking powder

2 tablespoons olive oil

8 ounces seitan, cut into ½-inch-thick "fingers"

Directions:

In a shallow dish, combine the flour, garlic powder, onion powder, cayenne, thyme, salt, and black pepper, whisking to mix thoroughly. In another shallow dish, whisk together the soy milk, lemon juice, and baking powder.

In a large sauté pan, heat the olive oil over medium-high heat until it shimmers. Dip each piece of seitan in the flour mixture, tapping off any excess flour. Next, dip the seitan in the soy milk mixture and then back in the flour mixture.

Fry until golden brown on each side, 3 to 4 minutes per side. Blot on paper towels before serving.

Nutrition:

Calories 447, Total Fat 11.1g, Total Carbohydrate 33g, Protein 48g

14. Sweet and Sour Tempeh

Preparation time: 10 minutes

Cooking time: 8 minutes

Servings: 4

Ingredients:

1 cup pineapple juice

1 tablespoon unseasoned rice vinegar

1 tablespoon soy sauce

1 tablespoon cornstarch

2 tablespoons coconut oil

1 pound tempeh, cut into thin strips

6 green onions (white and green parts), cut into strips

1 green bell pepper, diced

4 garlic cloves, minced

2 cups prepared brown or white rice

Directions:

In a small bowl, whisk together the pineapple juice, rice vinegar, soy sauce, and cornstarch and set aside.

In a wok or large sauté pan, heat the coconut oil over medium-high heat until it shimmers. Add the tempeh, green onions, and bell pepper and cook until vegetables soften, about 5 minutes.

Add the garlic and cook until it is fragrant, about 30 seconds. Add the sauce and cook until it thickens, about 3 minutes. Serve over rice.

Nutrition:

Calories 679, Total Fat 20g, Total Carbohydrate 100g, Protein 29g

15. Rigatoni with Roasted-Tomatoes and Arugula

Preparation time: 5 minutes

Cooking time: 5 minutes

Servings: 3

Ingredients:

1 pint cherry tomatoes

3 shallots, thinly sliced

sea salt

freshly ground black pepper

3 tablespoons extra virgin olive oil

one 9-ounce box rigatoni pasta

3 cloves garlic, minced

3 tablespoons red wine vinegar

4 ounces green olives, halved

¼ teaspoon red pepper flakes

2 cups baby arugula

Directions:

Preheat the oven to 400°F.

Bring a large pot of water to boil over high heat.

In a large ovenproof sauté pan, place cherry tomatoes and shallots in a single layer. Season to taste with sea salt and black pepper and drizzle with the olive oil. Put the pan in the preheated oven and cook for 20 minutes, until the tomatoes and shallots are soft.

Meanwhile, add the rigatoni to the boiling water. Cook according to the package directions until the pasta is al dente, nine to twelve minutes. Drain the pasta.

When the tomatoes and shallots are done roasting, move the pan to the stovetop and turn the stove on medium-high. Be careful not to touch the handle of the pan without a potholder.

Add the garlic to the pan and cook, stirring constantly, until it is fragrant, about 30 seconds.

Add the red wine vinegar and olives to the pan, using the side of the spoon to scrape any browned bits from the bottom of the pan. Bring to a simmer and stir in the red pepper flakes.

Toss the vegetables with the pasta, stirring in the arugula, which will wilt slightly from the heat. Serve immediately.

Nutrition:

Calories 145, Total Fat 3g, Total Carbohydrate 25g, Protein 5.3g

16. Spicy Nut-Butter Noodles

Preparation time: 15 minutes

Cooking time: 15 minutes

Servings: 4

Ingredients:

1 package soba noodles

½ cup vegetable stock

1 tablespoon minced fresh ginger

2 garlic cloves, minced

¼ cup soy sauce

¼ cup peanut butter or other nut butter

1 teaspoon sriracha or chili paste

4 green onions (white and green parts), chopped

chopped peanuts (optional)

Directions:

Prepare the soba noodles according to package directions. Drain and set aside.

In a small saucepan, combine the vegetable stock, ginger, garlic, soy sauce, peanut butter, and Sriracha, over medium-high heat, stirring until the peanut butter is melted and the sauce is heated through.

Toss the sauce with the hot noodles. Top with chopped green onions and peanuts, if using. Serve immediately.

Nutrition:18

Calories 165, Total Fat 8.4g, Total Carbohydrate g, Protein 8g

17. A.M. Breakfast Scramble

Preparation Time: 5 minutes

Cooking Time: 15 minutes

Servings: 2

Ingredients:

1 (14-ounce) package firm or extra-firm tofu

4 ounces mushrooms, sliced

½ bell pepper, diced

2 tablespoons nutritional yeast

1 tablespoon vegetable broth or water

½ teaspoon garlic powder

½ teaspoon onion powder

⅛ teaspoon freshly ground black pepper

1 cup fresh spinach

Directions:

Heat a large skillet over medium-low heat.

Drain the tofu, then place it in the skillet and mash it down with a fork

or mixing spoon. Stir in the mushrooms, bell pepper, nutritional yeast,

broth, garlic powder, onion powder, and pepper. Cover and cook for

10 minutes, stirring once after about 5 minutes.

Uncover, and stir in the spinach. Cook for an additional 5 minutes before serving.

Nutrition:

Calories: 230

Total Fat: 10g

Carbohydrates: 16g

Fiber: 7g

Protein: 27g

18. Loaded Breakfast Burrito

Preparation Time: 5 minutes

Cooking Time: 20 minutes

Servings: 2

Ingredients:

½ block (7 ounces) firm tofu

2 medium potatoes, cut into ¼-inch dice

1 cup cooked black beans (see here), drained and rinsed

4 ounces mushrooms, sliced

1 jalapeño, seeded and diced

2 tablespoons vegetable broth or water

1 tablespoon nutritional yeast

½ teaspoon garlic powder

½ teaspoon onion powder

¼ cup salsa

6 corn tortillas

Directions:

Heat a large skillet over medium-low heat.

Drain the tofu, then place it in the pan and mash it down with a fork or mixing spoon.

Stir the potatoes, black beans, mushrooms, jalapeño, broth, nutritional yeast, garlic powder, and onion powder into the skillet. Reduce the heat to low, cover, and cook for 10 minutes, or until the potatoes can be easily pierced with a fork.

Uncover, and stir in the salsa. Cook for 5 minutes, stirring every other minute.

Warm the tortillas in a microwave for 15 to 30 seconds or in a warm oven until soft.

Remove the pan from the heat, place one-sixth of the filling in the center of each tortilla, and roll the tortillas into burritos before serving.

Nutrition:

Calories: 535

Total Fat: 8g

Carbohydrates: 95g

Fiber: 21g

Protein: 29g

19. Southwest Sweet Potato Skillet

Preparation Time: 5 minutes

Cooking Time: 15 minutes

Servings: 4

Ingredients:

4 medium sweet potatoes, cut into ½-inch dice

8 ounces mushrooms, sliced

1 bell pepper, diced

1 sweet onion, diced

1 cup vegetable broth or water, plus 1 to 2 tablespoons more if needed

1 teaspoon garlic powder

½ teaspoon ground cumin

½ teaspoon chili powder

⅛ teaspoon freshly ground black pepper

Directions:

Heat a large skillet over medium-low heat.

When the skillet is hot, put the sweet potatoes, mushrooms, bell pepper, onion, broth, garlic powder, cumin, chili powder, and pepper in it and stir. Cover and cook for 10 minutes, or until the sweet potatoes are easily pierced with a fork.

Uncover, and give the mixture a good stir. (If any of the contents are beginning to stick to the bottom of the pan, add 1 to 2 tablespoons of broth.)

Cook, uncovered, for an additional 5 minutes, stirring once after about 2½ minutes, and serve.

Nutrition:

Calories: 158

Total Fat: 1g

Carbohydrates: 34g

Fiber: 6g

Protein: 6g

20. Peach Quinoa Porridge

Preparation Time: 10 minutes

Cooking Time: 20 minutes

Servings: 2

Ingredients:

¼ cup quinoa

¼ cup porridge oats

4 cardamom pods

1 cup unsweetened almond milk

2 ripe peaches, cut into slices

1 teaspoon maple syrup

Directions:

In a saucepan, add oats, cardamom pods, quinoa, water and almond milk and cook for 20 minutes on a simmer.

Discard the cardamom pods and add peaches and maple syrup.

Nutrition: Calories 361 Total Fat 16.3 g Saturated Fat 4.9 g

Cholesterol 114 mg Sodium 515 mg Total Carbs 29.3 g

Fiber 0.1 g Sugar 18.2 g

Protein 3.3 g

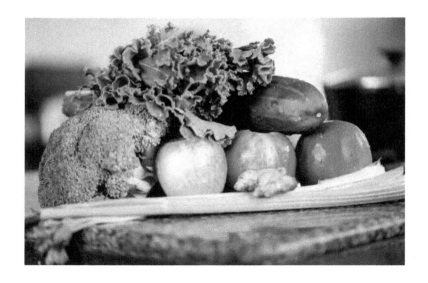

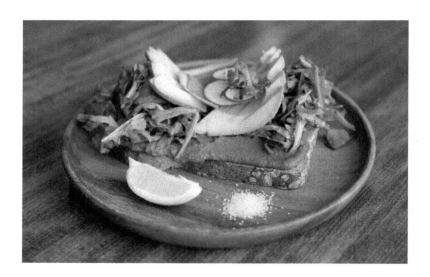

Chapter 2. : Salads, Soups, and Sides

21. Sautéed Collard Greens

Preparation Time: 10 minutes

Cooking Time: 25 minutes

Servings: 4

Ingredients:

1½ pounds collard greens

1 cup vegetable broth

½ teaspoon garlic powder

½ teaspoon onion powder

⅛ teaspoon freshly ground black pepper

Directions:

Remove the hard middle stems from the greens, then roughly chop the leaves into 2-inch pieces.

In a large saucepan, mix together the vegetable broth, garlic powder, onion powder, and pepper. Bring to a boil over medium-high heat, then add the chopped greens. Reduce the heat to low, and cover.

Cook for 20 minutes, stirring well every 4 to 5 minutes, and serve. (If you notice that the liquid has completely evaporated and the greens are beginning to stick to the bottom of the pan, stir in a few extra tablespoons of vegetable broth or water.)

Nutrition:

Calories: 28

Total Fat: 1g

Carbohydrates: 4g

Fiber: 2g

Protein: 3g

22. Crispy Cauliflower Wings

Preparation Time: 10 minutes

Cooking Time: 40 minutes

Servings: 6

Ingredients:

1 cup oat milk (here)

¾ cup gluten-free or whole-wheat flour

2 teaspoons garlic powder

2 teaspoons onion powder

½ teaspoon paprika

¼ teaspoon freshly ground black pepper

1 head cauliflower, cut into bite-size florets

Directions:

Preheat the oven to 425°F. Line a baking sheet with parchment paper.

In a large bowl, whisk together the milk, flour, garlic powder, onion powder, paprika, and pepper. Add the cauliflower florets, and mix until the florets are completely coated.

Place the coated florets on the baking sheet in an even layer, and bake for 40 minutes, or until golden brown and crispy, turning once halfway through the cooking process. Serve.

Nutrition:

Calories: 96

Total Fat: 1g

Carbohydrates: 20g

Fiber: 2g

Protein: 3g

23. Baked Taquitos with Fat-Free Refried Beans

Preparation Time: 5 minutes

Cooking Time: 25 minutes

Servings: 4

Ingredients:

2 cups pinto beans, cooked (see here)

1 teaspoon chili powder

1 teaspoon ground cumin

½ teaspoon garlic powder

½ teaspoon onion powder

¼ teaspoon red pepper flakes

12 corn tortillas

Directions:

Preheat the oven to 400°F. Line a baking sheet with parchment paper.

Combine the beans, chili powder, cumin, garlic powder, onion powder, and red pepper flakes in a food processor or blender. Pulse or blend on low for 30 seconds, or until smooth, then set aside.

Place the tortillas on the baking sheet, and bake for 1 to 2 minutes. This helps soften the tortillas and makes rolling them much easier.

Remove the tortillas from the oven, then add a couple of heaping tablespoons of the refried beans to the bottom half of each corn tortilla. Roll the tortillas tightly, and place them back on the baking sheet, seam-side down.

Bake for 20 minutes, turning once after about 10 minutes, and serve.

Nutrition:

Calories: 286

Total Fat: 3g

Carbohydrates: 56g

Fiber: 13g

Protein: 12g

24. 15-Minute French Fries

Preparation Time: 10 minutes

Cooking Time: 1 hour

Servings: 6

Ingredients:

2 pounds medium white potatoes

1 to 2 tablespoons no-salt seasoning

Directions:

Preheat the oven to 400°F. Line a baking sheet with parchment paper.

Wash and scrub the potatoes, then place them on the baking sheet and bake for 45 minutes, or until easily pierced with a fork.

Remove the potatoes from the oven, and allow to cool in the refrigerator for about 30 minutes, or until you're ready to make a batch of fries.

Preheat the oven to 425°F. Line a baking sheet with parchment paper.

Slice the cooled potatoes into the shape of wedges or fries, then toss them in a large bowl with the no-salt seasoning.

Spread the coated fries out in an even layer on the baking sheet. Bake for about 7 minutes, then remove from the oven, flip the fries over, and redistribute them in an even layer. Bake for another 8 minutes, or until the fries are crisp and golden brown, and serve.

Nutrition:

Calories: 104

Total Fat: 0g

Carbohydrates: 24g

Fiber: 4g

Protein: 3g

25. Fluffy Mashed Potatoes with Gravy

Preparation Time: 10 minutes

Cooking Time: 15 minutes

Servings: 6

Ingredients:

FOR THE MASHED POTATOES

8 red or Yukon Gold potatoes, cut into 1-inch cubes

½ cup plant-based milk (here or here)

1 teaspoon garlic powder

1 teaspoon onion powder

FOR THE GRAVY

2 cups vegetable broth, divided

¼ cup gluten-free or whole-wheat flour

½ teaspoon garlic powder ½ teaspoon onion powder

¼ teaspoon freshly ground black pepper

¼ teaspoon dried thyme

¼ teaspoon dried sage

Directions:

Bring a large stockpot of water to a boil over high heat, then gently and carefully immerse the potatoes. Cover, reduce the heat to medium, and boil for 15 minutes, or until the potatoes are easily pierced with a fork.

Drain the liquid, and return the potatoes to the pot. Using a potato masher or large mixing spoon, mash the potatoes until smooth.

Stir in the milk, garlic powder, and onion powder.

Meanwhile, in a medium saucepan, whisk together ½ cup of broth and the flour. Once no dry flour is left, whisk in the remaining 1½ cups of broth.

Stir in the garlic powder, onion powder, pepper, thyme, and sage. Bring the gravy to a boil over medium-high heat, then reduce the heat to low.

Simmer for 10 minutes, stirring every other minute, and serve with the mashed potatoes.

Nutrition:

Calories: 260 Total Fat: 1g

Carbohydrates: 56g

Fiber: 4g

Protein: 8g

Chapter 3. : Entrées

26. Black Bean and Quinoa Salad

Preparation Time: 10 minutes Cooking Time: 0 minutes

Servings: 10

Ingredients:

15 ounces cooked black beans

1 medium red bell pepper, cored, chopped

1 cup quinoa, cooked

1 medium green bell pepper, cored, chopped

1/2 cup vegan feta cheese, crumbled

Directions:

Place all the ingredients in a large bowl, except for cheese, and stir until incorporated.

Top the salad with cheese and serve straight away.

Nutrition: Calories: 64 Fat: 1 g Carbs: 8 g

Protein: 3 g

Fiber: 3 g

27. Grilled Zucchini with Tomato Salsa

Preparation Time: 10 minutes

Cooking Time: 8 minutes

Servings: 4

Ingredients:

4 zucchinis, sliced 1 tbsp. Olive oil Salt and pepper to taste

1 cup tomatoes, chopped 1 tbsp. Mint, chopped

1 tsp. Red wine vinegar

Directions:

Preheat your grill.

Coat the zucchini with oil and season with salt and pepper.

Grill for 4 minutes per side.

Mix the remaining ingredients in a bowl.

Top the grilled zucchini with the minty salsa.

Nutrition:

Calories 71 Total fat 5 g Saturated fat 1 g

Cholesterol 0 mg Sodium 157 mg Total carbohydrate 6 g

Dietary fiber 2 g Protein 2 g Total sugars 4 g

Potassium 413 mg

28. Eggplant Parmesan

Preparation Time: 20 minutes Cooking Time: 1 hour

Servings: 8

Ingredients:

Cooking spray

2 eggplants, sliced into rounds

Salt and pepper to taste

2 tbsp. Olive oil

1 cup onion, chopped

2 cloves garlic, crushed and minced

28 oz. Crushed tomatoes

¼ cup red wine

1 tsp. Dried basil

1 tsp. Dried oregano

½ cup parmesan cheese

1 cup mozzarella cheese Basil leaves, chopped

Directions:

Preheat your oven to 400 degrees f.

Spray your baking pan with oil.

Arrange the eggplant in the baking pan.

Season with salt and pepper.

Roast for 20 minutes.

In a pan over medium heat, add the oil and cook the onion for 4 minutes.

Add the garlic and cook for 1 to 2 minutes.

Stir in the rest of the ingredients except the cheese and basil.

Simmer for 10 minutes.

Spread the sauce on a baking dish.

Top with the eggplant slices.

Sprinkle the mozzarella and parmesan on top.

Bake in the oven for 25 minutes.

Nutrition:

Calories 192

Total fat 9 g   Saturated fat 4 g   Cholesterol 18 mg

Sodium 453 mg   Total carbohydrate 16 g

Dietary fiber 5 g   Protein 10 g

Total sugars 8 g   Potassium 632 mg

29. Coconut Chickpea Curry

Preparation Time: 10 minutes

Cooking Time: 30 minutes

Servings: 4

Ingredients:

2 teaspoons coconut flour

16 ounces cooked chickpeas

14 ounces tomatoes, diced

1 large red onion, sliced

1 ½ teaspoon minced garlic

½ teaspoon of sea salt

1 teaspoon curry powder

1/3 teaspoon ground black pepper

1 ½ tablespoons garam masala

1/4 teaspoon cumin 1 small lime, juiced

13.5 ounces coconut milk, unsweetened

2 tablespoons coconut oil

Directions:

Take a large pot, place it over medium-high heat, add oil and when it melts, add onions and tomatoes, season with salt and black pepper and cook for 5 minutes.

Switch heat to medium-low level, cook for 10 minutes until tomatoes have released their liquid, then add chickpeas and stir in garlic, curry powder, garam masala, and cumin until combined.

Stir in milk and flour, bring the mixture to boil, then switch heat to medium heat and simmer the curry for 12 minutes until cooked.

Taste to adjust seasoning, drizzle with lime juice, and serve.

Nutrition:

Calories: 225

Fat: 9.4 g

Carbs: 28.5 g

Protein: 7.3 g

Fiber: 9 g

30. Mediterranean Chickpea Casserole

Preparation Time: 10 minutes Cooking Time: 60 minutes

Servings: 4

Ingredients:

3 cups baby spinach

2 medium red onions, peeled, diced

2 1/2 cups tomatoes

3 cups cooked chickpeas

1 ½ teaspoon minced garlic

1/3 teaspoon ground black pepper

1 ¼ teaspoon salt

1/4 teaspoon allspice

1 tablespoon coconut sugar

1 teaspoon dried oregano

1/4 teaspoon cayenne

1/4 teaspoon cloves 2 bay leaves

1 tablespoon coconut oil

2 tablespoons olive oil

1 cup vegetable stock

1 lemon, juiced

2 ounces vegan feta cheese

Directions:

Take a large skillet pan, place it over medium-high heat, add coconut oil and when it melts, add onion and cook for 5 minutes until softened.

Switch heat to medium-low level, stir in garlic, cook for 2 minutes, then stir in tomatoes, add all the spices and bay leaves, pour in the stock, stir until mixed and cook for 20 minutes.

Then stir in chickpeas, simmer cooking for 15 minutes until the cooking liquid has reduced by one-third, stir in spinach and cook for 3 minutes until it begins to wilt.

Then stir in olive oil, sugar and lemon juice, taste to adjust seasoning, and remove and discard bay leaves.

When done, top chickpeas with cheese, broil for 5 minutes until cheese has melted and golden brown, then garnish with parsley and

Nutrition:

Calories: 257.8 Fat: 3.8 g Carbs: 47.1 g Protein: 10.3 g

Fiber: 9.4 g

31. Sweet Potato and White Bean Skillet

Preparation Time: 10 minutes

Cooking Time: 45 minutes

Servings: 4

Ingredients:

1 large bunch of kale, chopped

2 large sweet potatoes, peeled, ¼-inch cubes

12 ounces cannellini beans

1 small onion, peeled, diced

1/8 teaspoon red pepper flakes

1 teaspoon salt

1 teaspoon cumin

½ teaspoon ground black pepper

1 teaspoon curry powder

1 1/2 tablespoons coconut oil

6 ounces coconut milk, unsweetened

Directions:

Take a large skillet pan, place it over medium heat, add ½ tablespoon oil and when it melts, add onion and cook for 5 minutes.

Then stir in sweet potatoes, stir well, cook for 5 minutes, then season with all the spices, cook for 1 minute and remove the pan from heat.

Take another pan, add remaining oil in it, place it over medium heat and when oil melts, add kale, season with some salt and black pepper, stir well, pour in the milk and cook for 15 minutes until tender.

Then add beans, beans, and red pepper, stir until mixed and cook for 5 minutes until hot.

Serve straight away.

Nutrition:

Calories: 263

Fat: 4 g

Carbs: 44 g

Protein: 13 g

Fiber: 12 g

32. Kung Pao Brussels Sprouts

Preparation Time: 10 minutes

Cooking Time: 25 minutes

Servings: 1

Ingredients:

2 pounds brussels sprouts, halved

1 teaspoon minced garlic

¾ teaspoon ground black pepper

1 tablespoon cornstarch

1 ½ teaspoon salt

1 tablespoon brown sugar

1/8 teaspoon red pepper flakes

1 tablespoon sesame oil

2 tablespoons olive oil

2 teaspoons apple cider vinegar

1/2 cup soy sauce 1 tablespoon hoisin sauce

2 teaspoons garlic chili sauce

1/2 cup water

Sesame seeds as needed for garnish

Green onions as needed for garnish

Chopped roasted peanuts as needed for garnish

Directions:

Place sprouts on a baking sheet, drizzle with oil, season with salt and black pepper, and then bake for 20 minutes at 425 degrees f until crispy and tender.

Meanwhile, take a skillet pan, place it over medium heat, add oil and when hot, add garlic and cook for 1 minute until fragrant.

Then stir in cornstarch and remaining ingredients, except for garnishing ingredients and simmer for 3 minutes, set aside until required.

When brussel sprouts have roasted, add them to the sauce, toss until mixed and broil for 5 minutes until glazed.

When done, garnish with nuts, sesame seeds, and green onions and then serve.

Nutrition:

Calories: 272 Fat: 17 g Carbs: 26 g Protein: 10 g

Fiber: 7 g

33. Artichoke White Bean Sandwich Spread

Preparation Time: 10 minutes

Cooking Time: 0 minutes

Servings: 4

Ingredients:

½ cup raw cashews, chopped

Water

1 clove garlic, cut into half

1 tablespoon lemon zest

1 teaspoon fresh rosemary, chopped

¼ teaspoon salt

¼ teaspoon pepper

6 tablespoons almond

1 15.5-ounce can cannellini beans, rinsed and drained well

3 to 4 canned artichoke hearts, chopped

¼ cup hulled sunflower seeds

Green onions, chopped, for garnish

Directions:

Soak the raw cashews for 15 minutes in enough water to cover them.

Drain and dab with a paper towel to make them as dry as possible.

Transfer the cashews to a blender and add the garlic, lemon zest, rosemary, salt and pepper. Pulse to break everything up and then add the milk, one tablespoon at a time, until the mixture is smooth and creamy.

Mash the beans in a bowl with a fork. Add the artichoke hearts and sunflower seeds. Toss to mix.

Pour the cashew mixture on top and season with more salt and pepper if desired. Mix the ingredients well and spread on whole-wheat bread, crackers, or a wrap.

Nutrition:

Calories 200

Fats 4 g

Carbohydrates 39 g

Proteins 8 g

Chapter 4. : Smoothies and

Beverages

34. Cold-Brew Peach Iced Tea

Preparation Time: 10 minutes

Cooking Time: 0 minutes

Servings: 6

Ingredients:

4 ripe peaches, sliced

8 cups water

5 tea bags (black, green, or white)

Directions:

In a pitcher, combine the peach slices, water, and tea bags. Place in the refrigerator, and allow to steep overnight (8 to 12 hours). Store in the refrigerator for up to 5 days.

Nutrition:

Calories: 39 Total Fat: 0g Carbohydrates: 9g Fiber: 2g Protein: 1g

35. Maple-Cinnamon Latte

Preparation Time: 5 minutes

Cooking Time: 0 minutes

Servings: 2

Ingredients:

3 cups plant-based milk (here or here)

1 tablespoon maple syrup

1 teaspoon ground cinnamon

Directions:

In a medium saucepan on the stovetop, heat the milk until it just begins to boil, or microwave in a microwave-safe bowl on high for 2 minutes.

Pour the warmed milk, maple syrup, and cinnamon into a blender, and blend for 1 to 2 minutes, or until the mixture turns frothy. Serve warm.

Nutrition:

Calories: 89 Total Fat: 5g Carbohydrates: 11g Fiber: 2g

Protein: 2g

36. Apple Pie Smoothie

Preparation Time: 5 minutes Cooking Time: 0 minutes

Servings: 2

Ingredients:

1 large green apple, peeled and cored

¼ cup raspberries

¼ teaspoon cinnamon

⅛ teaspoon nutmeg

1 cup spinach 1 tablespoon of chia seeds

1 teaspoon vanilla extract

1 cup unsweetened almond milk

Directions:

Add all ingredients to a blender and blend until a smooth consistency is achieved. Serve immediately.

Nutrition:

Total Fat: 6.1g   Cholesterol: 0mg   Sodium: 106mg   Total carbohydrates: 25.4g Dietary Fiber: 9.6g Protein: 3.8g

Calcium: 337mg Potassium: 374mg Iron: 3mg

Vitamin D: 1mcg

37. Exotic Kale Smoothie

Preparation Time: 5 minutes

Cooking Time: 0 minutes

Servings: 1

Ingredients:

1 cup mango, cubed

1 orange, peeled

1 cup cucumber, chopped

1 tablespoon flax seeds

1 cup kale, chopped

Directions:

Add all ingredients to a blender and blend until a smooth consistency is achieved. Serve immediately.

Nutrition:

Total Fat: 3.2g

Cholesterol: 0mg Sodium: 35mg Total carbohydrates: 59.1g

Dietary Fiber: 10.5g Protein: 7.1g Calcium: 200mg

Potassium: 1149mg

38. Ginger Tea

Preparation Time: 35 minutes

Cooking Time: 0 minutes

Servings: 1

Ingredients:

½ cup fresh ginger, sliced

3 cups water

1 tablespoon maple syrup

Directions:

Place the ground ginger and water in small saucepan. Bring to a boil over high heat. Reduce heat to medium and simmer for about 25 minutes.

Strain ginger slices. Can be discarded or reserved for another use. Stir in maple syrup and serve hot. Tea can be refrigerated and reheated if necessary.

Nutrition:

Total Fat: 2.6g Cholesterol: 0mg Sodium: 37mg

Total carbohydrates: 44g Dietary Fiber: 5.4g

Protein: 3.9g Calcium: 85mg

Chapter 5. : Snacks and Desserts

39. Chocolate fudge

Preparation Time: 10 minutes

Cooking Time: 0 minutes

Servings: 12

Ingredients:

4 oz unsweetened dark chocolate

3/4 cup coconut butter

15 drops liquid stevia 1 tsp vanilla extract

Directions:

Melt coconut butter and dark chocolate.

Add ingredients to the large bowl and combine well.

Pour mixture into a silicone loaf pan and place in refrigerator until set.

Cut into pieces and serve.

Nutrition:

Calories 157 Fat 14.1 g Carbohydrates 6.1 g Sugar 1 g

Protein 2.3 g Cholesterol 0 mg;

40. Quick chocó brownie

Preparation Time: 10 minutes

Cooking Time: 0 minutes

Servings: 1

Ingredients:

1/4 cup almond milk

1 tbsp cocoa powder

1 scoop chocolate protein powder

1/2 tsp baking powder

Directions:

In a microwave-safe mug blend together baking powder, protein powder, and cocoa.

Add almond milk in a mug and stir well.

Place mug in microwave and microwave for 30 seconds.

Serve and enjoy.

Nutrition:

Calories 207 Fat 15.8 g Carbohydrates 9.5 g Sugar 3.1 g Protein 12.4 g Cholesterol 20 mg;

41. Simple almond butter fudge

Preparation Time: 15 minutes

Cooking Time: 0 minutes

Servings: 8

Ingredients:

1/2 cup almond butter

15 drops liquid stevia

2 1/2 tbsp coconut oil

Directions:

Combine together almond butter and coconut oil in a saucepan.

Gently warm until melted.

Add stevia and stir well.

Pour mixture into the candy container and place in refrigerator until set.

Serve and enjoy.

Nutrition:

Calories 43 Fat 4.8 g Carbohydrates 0.2 g Protein 0.2 g

Sugars 0 g Cholesterol 0 mg;

42. **Chocolate and Avocado Pudding**

Preparation Time: 3 hours and 10 minutes Cooking Time: 0 minutes

Servings: 1

Ingredients:

1 small avocado, pitted, peeled 1 small banana, mashed

1/3 cup cocoa powder, unsweetened

1 tablespoon cacao nibs, unsweetened

1/4 cup maple syrup 1/3 cup coconut cream

Directions:

Add avocado in a food processor along with cream and then pulse for 2 minutes until smooth.

Add remaining ingredients, blend until mixed, and then tip the pudding in a container.

Cover the container with a plastic wrap; it should touch the pudding and refrigerate for 3 hours.

Serve straight away.

Nutrition: Calories: 87 Cal Fat: 7 g Carbs: 9 g Protein: 1.5 g

Fiber: 3.2 g

43. Chocolate Avocado Ice Cream

Preparation Time: 1 hour and 10 minutes

Cooking Time: 0 minutes Servings: 2

Ingredients:

4.5 ounces avocado, peeled, pitted

1/2 cup cocoa powder, unsweetened

1 tablespoon vanilla extract, unsweetened

1/2 cup and 2 tablespoons maple syrup

13.5 ounces coconut milk, unsweetened 1/2 cup water

Directions:

Add avocado in a food processor along with milk and then pulse for 2 minutes until smooth.

Add remaining ingredients, blend until mixed, and then tip the pudding in a freezer-proof container.

Place the container in a freezer and chill for freeze for 4 hours until firm, whisking every 20 minutes after 1 hour.

Nutrition:

Calories: 80.7 Cal Fat: 7.1 g Carbs: 6 g Protein: 0.6 g

Fiber: 2 g

44. Watermelon Mint Popsicles

Preparation Time: 8 hours and 5 minutes Cooking Time: 0 minute

Servings: 8

Ingredients:

20 mint leaves, diced 6 cups watermelon chunks

3 tablespoons lime juice

Directions:

Add watermelon in a food processor along with lime juice and then pulse for 15 seconds until smooth.

Pass the watermelon mixture through a strainer placed over a bowl, remove the seeds and then stir mint into the collected watermelon mixture.

Take eight Popsicle molds, pour in prepared watermelon mixture, and freeze for 2 hours until slightly firm.

Then insert popsicle sticks and continue freezing for 6 hours until solid. Serve straight away

Nutrition: Calories: 90 Cal Fat: 0 g

Carbs: 23 g Protein: 0 g

45. Mango Coconut Chia Pudding

Preparation Time: 2 hours and 5 minutes Cooking Time: 0 minute

Servings: 1

Ingredients:

1 medium mango, peeled, cubed

1/4 cup chia seeds 2 tablespoons coconut flakes

1 cup coconut milk, unsweetened

1 1/2 teaspoons maple syrup

Directions:

Take a bowl, place chia seeds in it, whisk in milk until combined, and then stir in maple syrup.

Cover the bowl with a plastic wrap; it should touch the pudding mixture and refrigerate for 2 hours until the pudding has set.

Then puree mango until smooth, top it evenly over pudding, sprinkle with coconut flakes and serve.

Nutrition:

Calories: 159 Cal Fat: 9 g Carbs: 17 g

Protein: 3 g

Fiber: 6 g

Chapter 6. : Sauces, Dressings, and

Dips

46. Spinach Dip

Preparation Time: 10 minutes

Cooking Time: 1 minutes

Servings: 14

Ingredients:

6 ounces spinach, wilted

3 tablespoons of oil

¾ of a yellow onion, diced

3 large garlic cloves, minced

¾ cup raw cashews, soaked

¾ block of soft tofu

½ teaspoon salt

Directions:

Sauté onion with oil in a pan over medium heat until soft.

Add the garlic and cook while stirring for 30 seconds.

Transfer the onion and garlic mixture to the blender.

Add spinach, cashews, tofu, and salt then blend until smooth.

Serve.

Nutrition:

Calories 16

Total Fat 1.1 g

Saturated Fat 0.4 g

Cholesterol 2 mg

Sodium 84 mg

Total Carbs 2.1 g

Sugar 1.3 g

Fiber 0.3 g

Protein 0.9 g

47. Lemon Dressing

Preparation Time: 5 minutes Cooking Time: 0 minutes

Servings: 6

Ingredients:

3 tablespoons lemon juice 2 tablespoons olive oil

2 cloves of minced garlic 1½ teaspoons Dijon mustard

½ teaspoon agave ½ teaspoon rice vinegar

¼ teaspoon salt Pepper to taste

Directions:

Add all the ingredients to a blender.

Press the pulse button and blend until it is lump free.

Serve.

Nutrition:

Calories 120 Total Fat 1.3 g

Saturated Fat 0.7 g Cholesterol 3 mg

Sodium 48 mg Total Carbs 1.8 g

Sugar 1.6 g

Fiber 0.1 g

Protein 0.2 g

48. Parsley Arugula Pesto

Preparation Time: 5 minutes Cooking Time: 0 minutes

Servings: 12

Ingredients:

1 clove garlic 1 cup parsley

1 cup arugula ¼ cup walnuts

¼ teaspoon salt 1 tablespoon olive oil

1 tablespoon lemon juice

Directions:

Add all the ingredients to a blender.

Press the pulse button and blend until it is lump free.

Serve.

Nutrition:

Calories 22 Total Fat 1.5 g

Saturated Fat 0.6 g Cholesterol 3 mg

Sodium 126 mg Total Carbs 6.3 g

Sugar 5.1 g   Fiber 0.7 g

Protein 0.6 g

49. Basil Peanut Salad Dressing

Preparation Time: 10 minutes Cooking Time: 0 minutes

Servings: 6

Ingredients:

3 cups basil leaves 1 cup peanuts

½ cup olive oil ¾ cup water

Juice from ½ of a lemon

1 pinch each of salt, pepper, red chili flakes, to taste

Directions:

Add all the ingredients to a blender.

Press the pulse button and blend until it is lump free.

Serve.

Nutrition:

Calories 86 Total Fat 1.8 g

Saturated Fat 0.8 g   Cholesterol 3 mg

Sodium 537 mg Total Carbs 7 g

Sugar 1.7 g

Fiber 0.5 g

Protein 4.6 g

50. Roasted Red Salsa

Preparation Time: 10 minutes Cooking Time: 0 minutes

Servings: 4

Ingredients:

½ yellow onion, quartered 4 ripe roma tomatoes, halved

1 jalapeno pepper, halved 3 cloves of garlic, peeled

1 tablespoon brown sugar ½ teaspoon salt

1 teaspoon apple cider vinegar

¼ cup fresh cilantro, chopped

Directions:

Add all the ingredients to a blender.

Press the pulse button and chop the ingredients into a chunky salsa.

Serve.

Nutrition:

Calories 93 Total Fat 0.2 g

Saturated Fat 0 g Cholesterol 0 mg

Sodium 738 mg Total Carbs 11.3 g

Sugar 0.2 g Fiber 0.5 g

Protein 0.3 g

Conclusion

Plants are a good source of all nutrients and minerals. They have low cholesterol, good lipids, and anti-oxidant characteristics which help to detoxify the body from pollutants. A plant-based diet has a significant impact on health, skin, and the environment. Plant-based diet improves and provides shine to the skin. I have observed my clear skin with a glow after the adoption of plant-based food in the first month. This book is a complete guide for beginners who intend to reduce weight, strengthen muscles and bones, and health-related problems such as heart diseases, obesity, and metabolic syndromes.

Enjoy this book with all vegan recipes which will help you to decide your daily food.

CPSIA information can be obtained
at www.ICGtesting.com
Printed in the USA
LVHW052019210621
690769LV00012B/1889